Monthly Cardio Activity Report Card

MONTHLY CARDIO ACTIVITY REPORT CARD

Name	ON TARGET DAYS
Date range: To	

1	January		/ 31	%
2	February		/	%
3	March		/ 31	%
4	April		/ 30	%
5	May		/ 31	%
6	June		/ 30	%
7	July		/ 31	%
8	August		/ 31	%
9	September		/ 30	%
10	October		/ 31	%
11	November		/ 30	%
12	December		/ 31	%

CHAPTER TWO

January

Cardio Activity - *Planned*

· 4 ·

Cardio Activity - *Completed for the month*

Notes/Reasons

January 20____

Days target achieved

31

Activity : *Cardio*

Target : *Minutes*

Include Step *count and / or* **Distance** *covered within each day. Also include any other metric if you want. If target achieved on a day then put a tick in the box.*

Monday	Tuesday	Wednesday	Thursday	Friday	Saturday	Sunday

Goals	Achievements

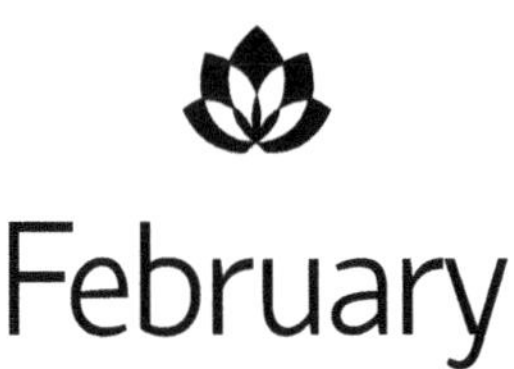

February

Cardio Activity - *Planned*

• 7 •

Cardio Activity - *Completed for the month*

Notes/Reasons

February 20_____

Days target achieved

2_

Activity: *Cardio*

Target : *Minutes*

Include Step *count and / or* **Distance** *covered within each day. Also include any other metric if you want. If target achieved on a day then put a tick in the box.*

Monday	Tuesday	Wednesday	Thursday	Friday	Saturday	Sunday

Goals	Achievements

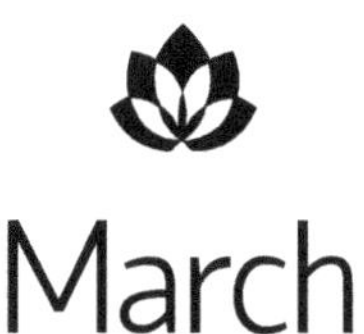

CHAPTER FOUR

March

Cardio Activity - *Planned*

Cardio Activity - *Completed for the month*

Notes/Reasons

March 20____

Days target achieved

31

Activity: *Cardio*

Target : *Minutes*

Include Step *count and / or* **Distance** *covered within each day. Also include any other metric if you want. If target achieved on a day then put a tick in the box.*

Monday	Tuesday	Wednesday	Thursday	Friday	Saturday	Sunday

Goals	Achievements

CHAPTER FIVE

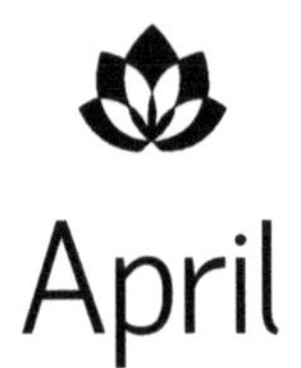

April

Cardio Activity - *Planned*

Cardio Activity - *Completed for the month*

Notes/Reasons

April 20_____

Activity: *Cardio*

Target : *Minutes*

Include Step *count and / or* **Distance** *covered within each day. Also include any other metric if you want. If target achieved on a day then put a tick in the box.*

Days target achieved

30

Monday	Tuesday	Wednesday	Thursday	Friday	Saturday	Sunday

Goals	Achievements

CHAPTER SIX

May

Cardio Activity - *Planned*

Cardio Activity - *Completed for the month*

Notes/Reasons

May 20____

Days target achieved

31

Activity : *Cardio*

Target : *Minutes*

Include Step *count and / or* **Distance** *covered within each day. Also include any other metric if you want. If target achieved on a day then put a tick in the box.*

Monday	Tuesday	Wednesday	Thursday	Friday	Saturday	Sunday

Goals	Achievements

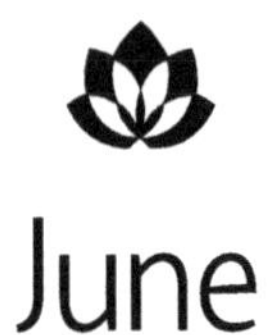

June

Cardio Activity - *Planned*

Cardio Activity - *Completed for the month*

Notes/Reasons

June 20____

Days target achieved

30

Activity : *Cardio*

Target : *Minutes*

Include Step count and / or **Distance** *covered within each day. Also include any other metric if you want. If target achieved on a day then put a tick in the box.*

Monday	Tuesday	Wednesday	Thursday	Friday	Saturday	Sunday

Goals	Achievements

CHAPTER EIGHT

July

Cardio Activity - *Planned*

Cardio Activity - *Completed for the month*

Notes/Reasons

July 20____

Activity: *Cardio*

Target : *Minutes*

Include Step count and / or **Distance** covered within each day. Also include any other metric if you want. If target achieved on a day then put a tick in the box.

Days target achieved

31

Monday	Tuesday	Wednesday	Thursday	Friday	Saturday	Sunday

Goals	Achievements

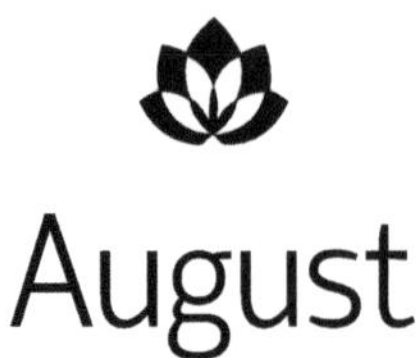

CHAPTER NINE

August

Cardio Activity - *Planned*

Cardio Activity - *Completed for the month*

Notes/Reasons

August 20____

Days target achieved

31

Activity: *Cardio*

Target : *Minutes*

Include Step *count and / or* **Distance** *covered within each day. Also include any other metric if you want. If target achieved on a day then put a tick in the box.*

Monday	Tuesday	Wednesday	Thursday	Friday	Saturday	Sunday

Goals	Achievements

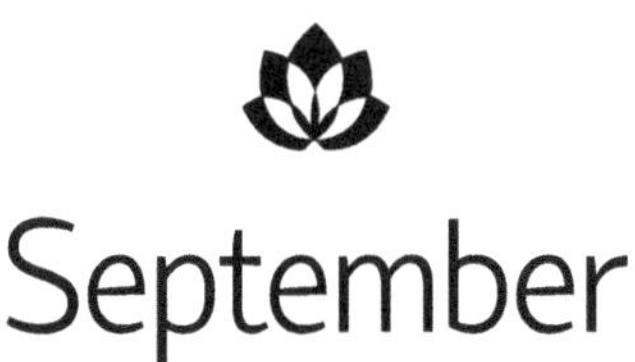

September

Cardio Activity - *Planned*

Cardio Activity - *Completed for the month*

Notes/Reasons

September 20____

Days target achieved

Activity : *Cardio*

Target : *Minutes*

Include Step *count and / or* **Distance** *covered within each day. Also include any other metric if you want. If target achieved on a day then put a tick in the box.*

30

Monday	Tuesday	Wednesday	Thursday	Friday	Saturday	Sunday

Goals	Achievements

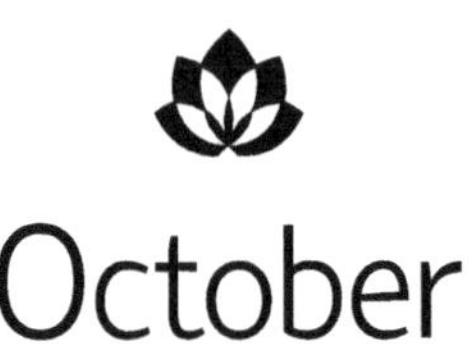

CHAPTER ELEVEN

October

Cardio Activity - *Planned*

• 31 •

Cardio Activity - *Completed for the month*

Notes/Reasons

October 20____

Activity: *Cardio*

Target : *Minutes*

Include Step *count and / or* **Distance** *covered within each day. Also include any other metric if you want. If target achieved on a day then put a tick in the box.*

Days target achieved

31

Monday	Tuesday	Wednesday	Thursday	Friday	Saturday	Sunday

Goals	Achievements

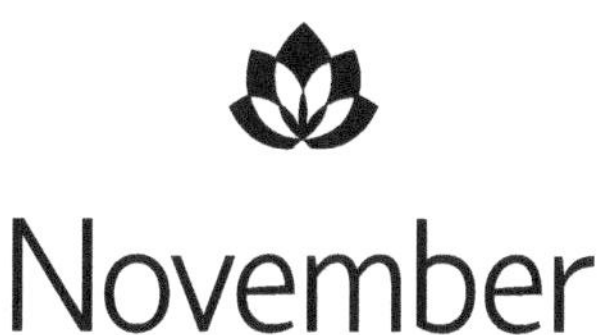

CHAPTER TWELVE

November

Cardio Activity - *Planned*

• 34 •

Cardio Activity - *Completed for the month*

Notes/Reasons

November 20____

Days target achieved

30

Activity : *Cardio*

Target : *Minutes*

Include Step *count and / or* **Distance** *covered within each day. Also include any other metric if you want. If target achieved on a day then put a tick in the box.*

Monday	Tuesday	Wednesday	Thursday	Friday	Saturday	Sunday

Goals	Achievements

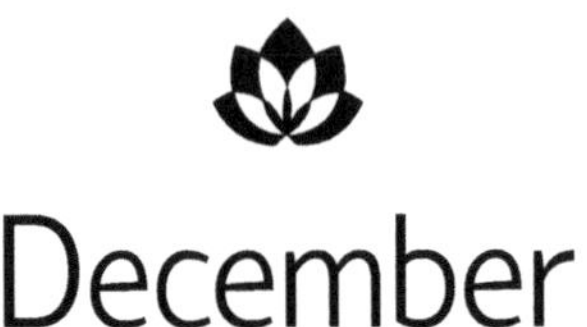

December

Cardio Activity - *Planned*

Cardio Activity - *Completed for the month*

Notes/Reasons

December *20____*

Days target achieved

31

Activity: *Cardio*

Target : *Minutes*

Include Step *count and / or* **Distance** *covered within each day. Also include any other metric if you want. If target achieved on a day then put a tick in the box.*

Monday	Tuesday	Wednesday	Thursday	Friday	Saturday	Sunday

Goals	Achievements

Reflections & Plan for next year

Please pen down your reflections for the year and also plan for next year.

www.ingramcontent.com/pod-product-compliance
Lightning Source LLC
Chambersburg PA
CBHW061146160726
48006CB00038B/2285